SIMPLE WAYS TO REMAIN HEALTHY

SOME PRACTICAL TIPS

Par Oum Jibril

CONTENTS

Preface   5

Introduction   7

Dedication   9

Reflection   11

Getting ready for change   13

Time Management   15

Let's Talk About Food!   17

Exercise   19

Stress   21

Being Grateful   23

Being Confident   25

 Unproductive Internet browsing   27

Patience   29

Life Is A Journey   31

Acceptance   33

Temptations   35

Good Character   37

Conclusion   39

CONTENTS

PREFACE

"In the name of the our Creator, The Most Gracious, The Most Merciful. All praise is due to Him - Lord of the Heavens and the Earth. We praise and Thank Him, and we seek His help and forgiveness for any wrong that we might have done, consciously or unconsciously. We seek His protection from any evil that might affect us, directly or indirectly. We also ask for His guidance, as whomever He guides, will never be misguided, and whomever He allows to go astray, will never be guided. We sincerely hope to be among those who enjoy a balanced, peaceful and healthy lifestyle in this life, and to be among the righteous ones in the Hereafter."

INTRODUCTION

It is my pleasure to share with you a few tips of what I have learnt through years of studies and research, as well as from my personal experience. Nowadays, most of us barely find the time to dedicate to important things in our lives, let alone having some time for ourselves. Our day seems to fly by without us getting much of stuffs done. Consequently, we are faced with an accumulation of tasks to accomplish, which definitely lead to a lot of stress and frustrations. No wonder, we are not as happy as we would want to be. These simple ways that I am going to share with you are only just a few tips from a lot more . I am sure that if you take the time to understand and reflect upon some of the tips, you will surely be able to give yourself, as well as your loved ones the quality lifestyle that you deserve and live happily ever after. So, without any more delay, let's get sarted!

DEDICATION

I would like to thank my parents-who are devoting their precious time to their children and grand-children, my siblings-without them I would not be who I am today, my husband-for his continuous love and support, my daughter- the gift of my life, and all those who has influenced my life positively-directly or indirectly. My greatest and sincere gratitude goes, without any doubt, to our Creator-without Whose intervention I would not be here today!

REFLECTION

Let us take a few minutes of our precious time for ourselves, so that we can reflect on our life. We deserve this "me" moment, even though we do not realise how important this is. If we do not take the time to help ourselves, no one else will. Let us ask this question: " Am I happy right now?", " How am I feeling right now?". If the answer to the first question is "no", then let us find out what aspect or aspects of our lives we are not happy about? We can write this down. We can do the same for any other feelings and try find out ways that we can change our situation, or what can be done for us to feel better. There are a lot of things that we cannot change in our lives, let alone changing people. People change only if there is a willingness to do so, otherwise, we can do everything in our power, but if that person does not internally want to change, we are just wasting our time and effort, and in addition getting frustrated in the process for nothing. However, if changes cannot happen, we can at least prepare ourselves better in order to face these challenges or issues. Hopefully, after dedicating some time reflecting on what is and what is not working in our lives, we can move on to the next step.

GETTING READY
FOR CHANGE

In order for changes or progress to happen we should be willing to take actions. To help us with this, we can ask this question – "Am I waking up every morning, excited to start my day, or am I all stressed and demotivated, doing what I am doing, because I have to do it and not because I want to do it? Everyone deserves to be happy. I am no exception." Only when we feel good about ourselves, will we be able to give our best, and thus having positive outcomes. In order to do this we have to understand and put ourselves first. Therefore, the most important and life-changing question is, "Am I ready to be happy?" If the answer is "yes", then the time for change starts now. We should be willing and ready to change our lives for the better. It all starts in our mind. It is a good idea to start a journal and write down our feelings and plans which can later be used as reference, and to remind us of our willingness to change, as we might get demotivated. We can write about our present feeling, how and why we would like to change. What are the things that we can do to make us feel good and what are the things that make us feel bad. Also, what are the things that we can or cannot change. This activity will also help us to see what are the possible options. We can try to visualise possible outcomes out of those possible options, if changes do occur. In the process, if we feel that we need to talk to someone that we can trust in order to see things more clearly, as well as have a second opinion, we can do so. That person can be a loved one, a friend or a

Oum Jibril

counselor.

TIME MANAGEMENT

Can we really manage time? We all have the same amount of time in a day. However, the key is how to use our time productively. We should plan and organise our time in advance. The best way to do this is to write down all the tasks that need to get done at least a day before. A "To-Do-List" is very helpful, which can later be adjusted accordingly. Another useful tip is to delegate some tasks to others, if possible, as this will reduce tasks that we have to do, but still get things done. A very effective way is to start our day earlier, which can be by waking up three hours before our usual wake-up time. If we really and badly want that positive change to happen, we have no other choice but to make this extra effort. Hence, we can proceed by putting the alarm three hours earlier, preferably far from our bed so that we are not tempted to sleep a little five minutes more, which can eventually turn into one hour more. The next thing that can help to wake us up is to have a glass of water ready by the bedside. At this point, it is very important to resist the urge of looking at our phone. We should remind ourselves that we have woken up earlier in order to provide ourselves with quality time to care for ourselves, so that we can be a more productive person. After using the bathroom, we can then do some light stretchings or exercise, dance if we wish, for about 20 minutes. This will boost up our body with oxygen, helping us to feel good physically, and we will be able to concentrate better. Then, we can sit in a comfortable position, away from our bed of course, closing our eyes, and telling ourselves:

"I am this beautiful person who is breathing in and out. I am feeding my body with fresh air. I can feel my heartbeats. My head, neck, arms, legs and my whole body, has been given to me by the Creator so that I am able to use them to move and function efficiently. I am grateful for this. I can feel the peace and positivity overflowing from within me. I am now ready to face the world"

We can say anything that we feel will make us feel better. After this exercise, we can look at our "To-Do-List" and re-arrange whatever needs to be done and according to priority. As mentionned before, delegating some tasks to some members of our family, if relevant, will allow us to have more time to do other important things that only we can do.

LET'S TALK ABOUT FOOD!

We cannot live without food. We all have our likes and dislikes about food, and there are certain foods that we prefer over others. Being healthy does not necessarily mean that we should stop eating foods that we like but are considered non-healthy. We should eat in the right amount, adjusting some ingredients wherever possible. We should also look at the portions. Like everything else, too little or too much are not good. We should adjust according to what our body needs. It is the same for people with medical conditions, like diabetes and hypertension. They need to control what they eat, but not to entirely stop, as this may lead to cravings and frustrations. The "why" and "how" and "when" to eat is very important in order to eat healthily. For example, in my early childhood, I have learnt that we should eat fruits as desserts, which is only after eating the main course meals. However, years later, I have learnt that it is best to eat fruits before the main course meals, as there are a lot of benefits and reasons to do so.

Research has shown that the best way to balance what we eat is to have one-third food, one-third water and one-third of space left in our stomach. How many times do we eat until we feel that we can no longer eat. Therefore, where is the space left for water and air?. It has been proved that having a glass of water before each meal helps to control how much we eat, in addition to hydrating our body for its optimal function. Moreover, having plenty of fruits and vegetables at home will help us to not indulge into too much of fast foods, although we know that we do want some fast food every now and then. We just have to make sure that we find ways to spend whatever excess calories we have taken, and stick to low carbohydrates meals and snacks. The secret is to always have a bottle of water, as well as plenty of fruits and vegetables, and snacks full of protein and fibre handy . In this way we will be able to avoid junk foods.

EXERCISE

There are all sorts of exercises that we can do on a daily basis. We do what we think and feel is best for us. Walking briskly for some time, and working out for at least twenty minutes per day, should be enough. Talk to a health professional if there are any medical conditions. However, walking is recommended as a safe exercise for everyone, even for pregnant women. Just remember to be safe. Dancing, cycling, jogging are other forms of exercises that will not affect daily routines drastically. Exercise can be done at any time during the day: after waking up, before going to school or work, during lunch time, or towards the end of the day. Like with everything else, you are the manager of your life, you know better than anyone else what is best for you. Therefore, arrange whatever you can around your schedule. If however you miss or cannot exercise everyday, you can do moderate to intense exercises, three times a week for forty-five to sixty minutes per session. Ensuring that you have enough sleep is also important, for our body to recover and heal. Life is simple if we keep it simple.

STRESS

One of the most common issues nowadays, is stress. Stress is a natural and unavoidable emotional state. We should bear in mind that a little stress now and then in our life is important in order to motivate us to progress and get things done. For example, if we are stressed about an exam, we will study. Nevertheless, like everything else, it is when we have an overdose of stress that things get out of control, thus affecting us not only physically, but also mentally, emotionally, as well as spiritually. With that said, what is the solution to stress? The best and easiest way is to keep ourselves away from stressful situations. If this is not possible for whatever reasons, we should at least get prepared to face stressful situations and events, or people, and look for ways to cope. Ask ourselves what has worked in the past and if we can use the same coping technique. We know that not all stressful situations can be avoided. We can write down what things, people or situations stress us, and we can then do what is best to make appropriate choices. Again, if we feel that there is a need to talk to someone we can trust, then we can do so.

BEING GRATEFUL

Being grateful for little and simple things help us to remain positive. Positive attracts positive. Let us be grateful for the organ called "heart" that has not stopped beating since it first started while we were still in the womb! Let us be grateful for the oxygen that we breath without which we will not be alive, and which we do not have to make the effort of buying or thinking about it. Let us also be grateful for the night and the day that alternates respectively, guiding us to be active and to rest accordingly. These are only some of the natural favors that happen to us, that we barely take the time to reflect upon, and to be grateful to our Creator for. We should also be grateful for our family, our home, our job and so much more. Just making it a habit to be grateful helps us to be happy with what we have, which in turn helps us to enjoy and respect our situation. Many things happen in our lives that we are not happy about. Instead of allowing those things or events to negatively affect our lives, let us take the positive lessons out of them. This will definitely remove a lot of stress from our lives and keep us happy.

BEING CONFIDENT

Self-confidence is very important if we want to be successful in life. We have to be confident in everything that we undertake in order to be successful. Confidence motivates us to move forward and to face challenges courageously. We cannot deny that life is full of challenges. However, it is by being confident that we can break barriers and make progress. If we do not feel confident enough to move forward, we need to work on it without delay so that we can achieve our goals sooner. There are a lot of lectures and information about self-confidence and personal development easily accessible on the internet nowadays. We can dedicate about half an hour to one hour of our time daily to search for materials that we think we need to work on, and concentrate and be consistent in this habit. No one knows us better than ourselves. We know what our strengths and weaknesses are. We can write them down, and work on strengthening ourselves, gaining the confidence that is required in order to become the better version of ourselves. No one else will do this for us but us. Therefore, we better get started and not waste any more time!

UNPRODUCTIVE INTERNET BROWSING

Undeniably, internet has made our lives a lot easier, be it on a personal, educational or professional basis. Without the internet we will not be able to achieve a lot nowadays. After a long day at school or a hard day at work we need to relax, and being on the net seems to be the easiest thing to do. We can socialise, watch movies and do a lot more on the net. However, some people are so addicted to the net that it is affecting all aspects of their life. Internet addiction is on the rise, especially with Facebook and Youtube. It should not be a problem if we are using the net productively. However, not being able to control and balance it's use can waste a lot of our precious time, and at the same time causing drastic problems in our life. One of big issues being the lack of communication among family members, among others. We should use the net for personal growth and development, and other productive ways.

PATIENCE

Being and remaining patient is easier said than done, especially in difficult situations. Most of us fail while waiting for the bus, or in a traffic jam. If only we could fly like birds! Everywhere we go, we have to wait in a queue for our turn. We have to be patient with our loved oned, especially with kids, we have to be patient while waiting for a job offer or for exam results. Almost everything in our daily life tests our patience. If we tell ourselves that whatever should happen will happen at the time that it is meant to happen, and that we do not always have control over certain things, our life will be a lot easier and less stressful. For example, wanting a parcel in earlier than we are supposed to receive it will only get us frustrated. Sunday will be here on Sunday, not before. While we are waiting, we can get ourselves occupied with other things that need to get done. Patience is the key to success. Whatever needs to happen will happen at the right time. Understanding this will save us, and allow us to concentrate on important things that are under our control. We just need to make the necessary effort and to wait patiently for the result.

LIFE IS A JOURNEY

Every second babies are born and people are dying throughout the world, regardless of age. Each and everyone of us who enters in this journey called life, has to leave at some point, as prescribed by the One who created us. Therefore, it is important to know the purpose of our existence in the first place, so that we can do what we need to do in order to make it through this journey successfully. If we do not follow the instructions of the Creator, who knows about His creation better than anyone else, then definitely we will make mistakes, which may have very serious consequences. Knowing that we are in this world for a fixed period of time, it is thus our responsibility to make each and every second worth living. If we had an argument with someone, let us forgive and move on with our life. We have nothing to lose. On the contrary, it is like leaving a burden behind which allows us to be free to move forward. Holding grudges is like a rope that ties us and prevents us from moving forward. Let us get rid of the rope and progress towards our goal. We do not have time to waste.

Let us stay positive, although I admit that this will be hard to do at times. At least we know that we have good intentions and we are giving it a try. One of the easiest ways to stay positive is to smile. Not only it makes us feel good internally, but considering that a smile is an act of charity, it does not cost us anything. On the contrary, it can make someone else's day. Many people find it hard to smile to people they know. Now, this becomes a lot harder with strangers. A smile can instantly make someone feel better. By feeling positive, we attract positiveness and repel what is negative. The state of positivity motivates us to achieve our objectives successfully and to share positivity to our surroundings. So, take along with us those who want to progress!

ACCEPTANCE

Like I said before, there are some things in life that we do not have any control over. We want someone to fall in love with us, we are trying very hard, doing whatever we can to attract that person, but we are not successful. We know that we have done our best, but it is still not working. Maybe there is something better for me, but I am too focused on what is not mine that I cannot see that something better is waiting for me. If something is meant to be, it will happen. If it is not meant to be, then we can waste our time, energy and happiness over it, it will neither not happen, or we might be successful temporarily. When it will break, it will be very hard to digest then. Therefore, it is better not to force things. Before doing something, we can meditate and ask our Creator if it is good for us. We will get the answer and then can proceed in what we need to do. Not everything tha we like is good for us, and not everything that we hate is bad for us. Sometimes, it is hard to accept reality, and it is hard to understand how things work. But we should learn to do things the correct way and accept the consequences of our actions.

TEMPTATIONS

This life is full of temptations: food, cars, houses, jewelleries, relationships...you name it. We may say that there are good temptations, hidden temptations and bad temptations. What tempts one person may not tempt someone else, and vice-versa. As it is, temptations come in different ways and forms. The first question that we should ask when faced with any doubt or temptation is, "Is this thing good for me and for my future, or I am going to get into trouble, feel guilty and ashamed afterwards?". We might get instant pleasure or satisfaction, but what about in the long run? Thinking twice or more, if required, will save us from doing something that we should not have to regret doing afterwards. We should trust our intuition. Most of the time, our intuition warns us if something is not right. What happens next is whether we have made the right decisions or not. Furthermore, we have to be ready to bear the consequences of our decisions. Some temptations are obvious, whereas those that are disguised and hidden will undoubtedly lead to deceptions. Thus, we have to be very careful and stay safe and out of trouble.

GOOD CHARACTER

Character is something that many of us do not really pay attention to but it is part of us, accompanying us all the time, whether we are conscious about it or not. What is good character? How would we like other people to describe us? Are we patient, easy to approach, friendly, and so one. We can learn and choose to have a good character. Kindness, righteousness and honesty are other examples of good characters. Character is like a garden. If we take good care of it, it will be productive. If we abandon it, wild grass will grow and take it over. At times we might give it some attention, but it is not well taken care of, some residual grass which will appear now and then.

Anger is one character trait that is often hard, but not impossible to control. If we try to understand ourselves and have the intentions to improve our character, we will not only feel good within ourselves, but we will feel more productive. Moreover, people will feel comfortable being in our presence, which will definitely improve our relationship with others.

CONCLUSION

I have only put a brief and general summary of simple things that we can apply in our daily life in order to be the better version of ourselves. Of course, individual needs may vary according to different aspects of our lives, whether it being physical, emotional, social or spiritual. I sincerely hope that you will benefit from this small piece of work. I will definitely share other tips with you that will contribute to a healthy lifestyle. Let us make the most out of this life journey! I wish you all the happiness, success, health and wealth of this world and the next!

The End

www.ingramcontent.com/pod-product-compliance
Lightning Source LLC
Chambersburg PA
CBHW051405280526
45784CB00007B/3109